Aftercare: Chemical Dependency Recovery

Book by the Author

A Path to Sobriety,
The Inside Passage
Volume I

A Path to Relapse Prevention,
The Inside Passage
Volume II

Aftercare: Chemical Dependency Recovery
The Inside Passage
Volume III

◊

Romancing San Francisco
[Volume I]

A Romance in Augsburg
[Volume II]

Where the Birds Don't Sing
[Volume III]

◊

Death on Demand
[Seven Suspenseful Short Stories]

Dracula's Ghost
[And Other Peculiar Stories]

✳

The Mumbler,
Murder by the Second Self

The Curse of the Viper Family
[The Abyss Virus Worm]
[To be released]

The Fruit Cake
[A Comedy-Tragedy]
[To be released]

*

Sirens
[Poems]

"After Eve"
[To be released]

What you need to know about Programming in Aftercare
For the Chemically Dependent

Aftercare: Chemical Dependency Recovery

✦

[The Inside Passage]
Volume III

----A Common Sense Book----
On Understanding the Elements of Growth,
Support and Healing

Dennis L. Siluk

iUniverse, Inc.
New York Lincoln Shanghai

Aftercare: Chemical Dependency Recovery
[The Inside Passage] Volume III

iUniverse, Inc.

For information address:
iUniverse, Inc.
2021 Pine Lake Road, Suite 100
Lincoln, NE 68512
www.iuniverse.com

ISBN: 0-595-30868-6

Printed in the United States of America

Dedicated: to those who have achieved sobriety, and are now working on non-use alternatives to life [Aftercare folks]…

Δ

"…there is rest and healing in the contemplation of antiquities."

—*Mark Twain*

Contents

◊

Acknowledgements

I want to thank my wife Rosa,
And Mother for their belief in me,
And now Papa Augusto, who said
Like my mother:
'God must have a plan for you.'

Note: There is much truth in what Mr. Mark Twain had to say in the above quote, and possible my reasoning being quite different than his, yet similar; therefore, I have always loved antiques, old coins, old rings, old everything. Old signatures, old books [First Editions],—they calm me, relax me, just like water does, especially as I walk along the rivers such as the Mississippi: in St. Paul, St. Louis, or New Orleans, as well as the Seine in Paris, or the Tames along the banks in London Town.

In addition, the spirit of the signatures come out, as my father-in-law has told me [whom is from Peru, 82-years old], to comfort me; whatever is the case, in both situations, and in paintings as well, I am always much more calm with them around, so there is truth in what Papa Augusto tells me, as there is healing in the waters, especially the flow of it. That goes for museums as well.

Now you may be asking: why am I bringing this up first hand, before I even get into the book? Good question. In recovery, a person needs to find what makes him tick [what triggers him, what calms him?] I just told you what calms me, along with traveling, and a good movie. Now you need to know for yourself.

Prelude

[The Inside Passage]

Aftercare is an element of prevention, with the ultimate goal for the individual to avoid a potential relapse. Aftercare is part of a circular form of continuing care, a cycle if you will, that includes ongoing assessments, suggestions, objectives and targets. It can be a group setting or for that matter, a one on one, with a counselor; most facilities offer both options.

The nature of Aftercare is more supportive than therapeutic, not quite like treatment, had you gone through it, this would be obvious. In Aftercare the counselor usually will present alternatives for using, growth, support. Simply put, helping you become the person you want to become. Since this is a book-format presentation, we will deal with Aftercare in a few different dimensions, that is, we can jump occasionally into a group setting, a one on one setting, a lecture setting, and so on. But first we just have to have a good idea of Aftercare, what it is, or what it should be. I have worked in the Chemical Dependency area going on 22-years, with another 22-years of usage, making my experience some 44-years in the making; and I am licensed in Minnesota, as of this writing [retiring]. And I've been certified in over ten countries to practice. I am now retiring from the field, and this most likely will be my last book on the subject of sobriety, prevention, addiction, treatment and aftercare. Incidentally this is my third book in the helping field of Alcoholism and Drugs, or better put, Chemical Dependency and Addiction.

Aftercare takes place, after treatment usually. Some of the segments in Aftercare, or at least the groups I have taught had assignments in reading, for meditation. Working on your personal inventory [your defects in character, or behavior you want to make changes to, that is, to make better oneself]. I often did lectures on urges [urges: meaning, something that seems like it is pushing you, insisting that you use, inside of you] and had the group members update me on how they were doing: the 'doing' part is called: 'hidden agendas', during the group processing session that is, and the group normally would give feedback if the client would ask for it [which I believe should be asked for and not forced upon the client]. In addition, I provided education in the way of movies, lectures, speakers, and the normal subjects I brought out in Aftercare, which we focused on, were for the most part, the: 12-step work, 12-traditions, relapse prevention, discussions on stresses the clients may be having [again, it is called hidden agendas—these uneasy, unsettled issues inside of you]; along with other chosen topics, such as triggers and symptoms. Affirmations were a big reminder for my clients also, a reminder in the sense of using them to build them back up, to rebuild self: love, regard, esteem. We must build ourselves up you know, we've been down too damn long.

And so, in this brief prelude, we look simply at the nature of the beast, so you do not get scared away. People often come to me and say:

"I've been through all the treatment, and now this, what is this all about..." In a like manner, AA can take the place of Aftercare if you wish, or become part of your Aftercare program. So Aftercare in a nutshell is simply 'Primary Prevention mixed with relapse prevention, dealing with a triangle of the continuing care cycle,' in the works: put another way, ongoing involvement with the continuum of care; and of course you need to be a non-user while in this arena.

This is also the time to look at the things you didn't have time to look at during treatment, but heard such as: physical dependence; or psychological dependence, or tolerance vs. cross tolerance vs cross addiction; a time to really dive into the broad spectrum of Chemical Dependency if you wish, or simply go for additional support while you're healing. By this time, you know what you need, and what you do not need; who you should be with, that is, hanging out with, or living with, and you also should know who is damaging to be with;—so get away from the negative ones, whoever they are.

Δ

A few phrases from the book: 'Denial…' a book written by, Sandi Bachom:

"Nobody ever thought I was a drunk until they had seen me sober."

"Alcoholism is the only disease that tries to convince you that you don't have it."

"Alcohol is patient; it will wait forever for us to return to it."

1

Terminology

For the most part, the Prelude explained the nature and makeup of Aftercare, as I understand it to be. And as it was run in all of my several programs at clinics and hospitals I've worked at; plus, I have helped in making up Aftercare programs for clinics as well. But for clarity sake, let me just go through it once more and into the first subject: or issue. First of all, I want to explain things in a form called: A) and B), ok? Then I will go directly to the terminology part which can be C). Furthermore, this book—for the most part—is being written for the layman, so he/she can look for what he/she needs, and at the same time, see what a program should look like. If it helps the professional, good, or the starting Counselor in this field, again, all the better; but it is the client that knows very little about what he/she is stepping into, and this should help them. No one really likes jumping into something they know very little about. You test the water to see if it is hot or cold. So here you go, see if you like it, it may be too hot or possible too cold for you, but whatever, it will not be a secret anymore.

A) The basic steps within the Aftercare session, is to:

1. The term: *Check in*, when in the group means: to update the group with your weekly activities. If you've had urges and or stress factors, this is the time to get them out; it can be called: getting out your hidden agendas,—you need to get it out so you and the group can go forward with a clear mind.

2. Hand in Assignments.

3. Break [we all need time to stand up, walk about, air our heads, especially if it is a 4-hour group].

4. Education/discussion. This is the area I will do a lecture, have a speaker in, or show a movie. After the event, there usually is a discussion on what you picked up out of this; or how it related to you, or could.

5. Closure. This is like the beginning, but shorter. Whereas, the *Check in* could take between 10 to 30 minutes, depending on 'hidden agendas,' the *closure* is usually ½ that time. You normally will bring out what lies ahead of you for the weekend, or week, and what you got out of the session.

B) Have a schedule for yourself, if you are a counselor that is. And if a client, here is what to expect from that schedule or itinerary [for the most part]:

1. The class is made up of, let's say the maximum amount of people to learn, don't exceed 13, beyond this, you are not giving what I consider good "Primary Prevention Aftercare", how can you, it will take forever just to get through the 'check in' and then break will come, and people get too worn out.

2. The reading is done, either by the counselor in a daily reader, or the AA Big Book, or the Red Book, on the 12-steps, and *Check In* has just finished also, now we go to either: finished hand outs from last session the client took home, or a lecture on, let's say 'depression,' or 'forgiveness,' or work on the 12-steps or 12-traditions, something like that.

3. Now you've taken your break, and as you return you will have a movie to watch, and make notes on, or [some people can not read or write, take this into consideration] give them your understanding on the issues involved with the movie, or the speaker's speech, or book reading the counselor may do, or have you do [you need a different approach with the folks that are a bit slower].

4. At this point we are next to Closure, but before you jump into this, you may want to do 'affirmations,' that is right, have everyone give everyone else a good build up, and themselves. An example might be, "Joe, you're really improving on opening up in class and sharing, you're becoming more assertive, and for myself, well, I'm just a good and nice guy now." Or you may give yourself another affirmation to the group that says: "I'm very proud of myself, I've told people for the first time, 'no' I didn't want to do this, when normally I'd say yes to appease them;" now the closure.

Now nothing is written in stone, and you can devise your own Aftercare group to match your cliental. These are simply examples, one of my examples that is, one that I used.

Terminology [understanding it]:

These terms are interchangeable with drugs or alcohol, yet they may have a brief difference in understanding.

1.   Physical Dependency vs. Psychological Dependency

Dependency means in essence, you are dependent on it. If you are an alcoholic, you are dependent on alcohol. If you are a heroin user, you are an addict, dependent on drug usage. The same goes for any drug. If you are an abuser, that means you have abused a drug or alcohol. Now listen up close, an abuser is not...I say not, necessarily a dependent, but a dependent is always an abuser. Does that make sense? If not, think about it. If you are a dependent, you have abused, and are abusing. Why, because you can't stop, and your body is craving for it, and you are abusing your body. Believe it or not, your abuse, dependence, your symptoms, sticks to everyone else, everyone around you. Now that we've got the two words out of the way, 'dependency,' and 'abuse,' let's go for the physical and psychological.

Physical vs. Psychological;—I will try and make this as painless and simple as I can, not for your sake necessarily, but mine. When I first looked at both of these, and I have a degree in psychology, I couldn't figure out in counseling school, why it was so hard for the teachers to simply come up with a simple way of explaining the difference. Too many PhD's out there trying to show off was my conclusion. Here it is in a nutshell:

   a.   Physical Dependency=symptoms of withdrawal, which can vary depending on the drug, amount used, and length of time used. Withdrawal in itself includes the physical body in revolt, it is poisoned, and it is fighting for your life, its life. Maybe I've oversimplified; possible so, therefore, let me add, if I have: it includes vomiting, cramps, convulsions, tremors, delirium, and can involve death. Let's move on to Psychological.

   b.   Psychological Dependence=in a nutshell again, should I try it? With all the psychology I've taken, I'm almost compelled to make it harder, but I can't: preoccupied. Now we can elaborate if you wish. Yes, in this psychological area the main word is preoccupation. Another way of putting it is compulsion, otherwise known as, impulse to continue the usage at any cost. Again, oversimplified, but to the point.

Now let's look at *Tolerance vs. Cross Tolerance*. You will hear these words in Treatment, Aftercare, Relapse Prevention classes, Chemical Dependency books, and you may not get a good break down of the terms, so you may want to read them over a few times. People will throw them around at AA, NA, GA, you know, all the support groups, either thinking you should know them, or bragging because they do, and you don't.

a.   Tolerance: it is a term used basically to imply, it takes more today to get me to the same point or high it had taken, or took: yesterday. Now let me get a little sophisticated, I don't usually, but I got to showoff some place: Let's use alcohol and heroin for our subjects in question. We could resort to using other forms of drugs, even over the counter drugs, or simply prescription drugs, but no—just, just alcohol and heroin will do for us. In these two drugs one can pinpoint what we talked about before, physical dependence, meaning, withdrawal [remember that word] have an effect on that person, if he/she does not get his or her fix; or if his or her tolerance level is not met.

b.   Cross Tolerance: it kind of speaks for itself, in that, we are talking now about more than one substance we are using. Again, this is in nature not a difficult term, but used often times quite loosely, and for the wrong reasons at times. Let me explain. Like the word Tolerance, without the 'cross' involved, which again implies, the need for higher doses to achieve an effect, one can quickly develop a tolerance to another drug, similar possible, with pharmacological action. The cells of the body are already conditioned to the other substance, consequently, the cross tolerance is simply combining drugs of similar nature. The person doing this is ripe for an overdose. If you are taking alcohol, don't take barbiturates, you got two sedatives in motion here, and this can be dangerous.

Now, we are coming to the end of Chapter One, it was short and quick chapter, like all the chapter in the book: but I do need to bring one more thing to your attention here. It is called 'Cross Addiction,' I left it for last simply because it would be easier for me to explain it now, and easier for you to learn it since you have the above information all tucked away in your brain. If you have Cross Tolerance, you mostly [I say most likely], have a cross addiction. Why do I say: "Most likely?" Because some drugs do not have a tolerance, but let's get back to the basics;—the reason a doctor or nurse asks you, "What is your drug history," is simply because, addiction to one drug sets up the body, or person involved, for addiction to similar drugs [pharmacologically]. We made it this far, now for Chapter two.

2

The Whole Person Concept

While you are reading this book you can do one of many things, as I can,—we can pretend we are in Aftercare, learning about Aftercare, or simply teaching Aftercare. I guess there is a forth option for me anyway, I can combine all of these together, and so I shall. You pick out what you want. But let's say we now are in the group, and I am going to give a lecture, and it is called: "The Whole Person Concept" and you are the client [counselors reading this, just read on, and listen, you're not the client].

Now one of the members of the group asks me:

"Why do we have to learn the concept you're about to lecture us?"

I say, "It is not a lecture for you to learn, it is one for me to present so you know where we're headed and what we should be doing in Aftercare," now he goes, "Hm…mm." And I'm ready to start.

The concept is simply, it knows who you are. That is it in a nutshell. No more, no less. But, and we all knew the 'but' was coming, there are several different areas. So the reason you are in Aftercare is to become a 'whole person,' again, you should be halfway there by now anyhow. Building yourself up is the secret in this concept: emotionally, mentally, socially and spiritually: along with, physically and working on the 'will'. My job as a counselor is to help you become the best person you can, in all of the above areas. I hope in the process you find the means in creating more energy and power in these areas.

Now what I am going to do is this: I tell the you [you being: the client], "…take a piece of paper, and what you need to do is write on it, or tell me how you are achieving this, 'whole person,' thing.'" And what you don't tell me is what we may need to work on. At the end of the road, I tell the client, "Take responsibility for your own behavior," that is what an adult does.

Now if I notice you have too much energy in the physical area being distributed, I may recommend you get some more in the mental area. Read more, go back to school [suggestions only]. And I may need for you to tell me how you plan on doing this. If you say, "I'm not going to," and it is not the reasonable thing to say, I say, "*adios amigo…*" school is over, no time for playing, only time for healing. You see, it doesn't happen by itself, we need team work here. We only take 'the willing.' Don't put the book down yet, if you do, simply go to the last chapter on 'Recovery,' read it and come back here.

We got to now go backwards, the client [you] has absorbed the information, and knows what has to be done, remember you are the client, for a little while anyway. What is back there that we left? It is called "Who am I?" We can achieve this by…wait, let me say, you may not like what you have to tell me, but you must, so we can go forward, ok, now back again, express your strengths, weaknesses, likes and dislikes about who you are [remember you are talking about yourself now]; give a bibliography account of you. What is most important in your life…this is who you are.

Now remember this is really a group exercise, although I've done it in one on one: Aftercare sessions with the Beau of Prisons, inmates, but in this field, you improvise if you have to, remember what I said before, "Whatever floats the boat," woops, I haven't used that expression yet—have I, but now I have. This Chapter has been short again, I know, but let's say: short and sweet is all that was needed,—now let's move on.

3

The Grieving Process

Before I get too far into this process of grieving, let me say, everyone healing, or recovering is grieving. You grieve what you have lost, and everyone grieves differently—some longer, others shorter periods of time. If it is a parent, you grieve. If it is an apartment, or house you've lived in for ten to sixteen-years, you grieve it; likewise, if it is a bottle of beer that you made love to for twenty-years or more you grieve it. If it is the high you left behind, you grieve it. If it is a spouse, a divorce, you grieve it. Grieving in a nutshell is letting go, while the wound heals. And in some cases it always leaves a scare, a reminder where you've been. And sometimes we open that wound—or the scare reopens itself when a person can't let go and go forward in his or her life. Yes: sad is still sad, and love is still love, and hate is still hate, and it's our old usage history that reminds us sometimes, and sometimes for very long periods time, of our past. But that is part of being human; having said that, we need to get on with the 'process.'

In an Aftercare session, this would be a lecture most likely, and could be a take home assignment, possible in a book to be read, or hand out literature to be reviewed, etc. If we were to translate this into the 'Whole Person Concept,' it may fall under emotional-psychological, or the spiritual-social, or even the mental-will category, or possible a combination.

1) First let's look at the word: Grief=mental suffering or distress, a loss.

2) We are giving up something; it could be based on retirement, possessions, food, moving, and of course, drugs and alcohol.

3) We have to face the main character called: denial, which equals="It is not so, not true." In alcohol usage, the person denies he/she has a problem.

In the grieving process:

4) We have to face: Anger, which one may say, "I am so very crazy…mad, angry." We ask the 'why' questions, we become angry at others, ourselves, and life in

general. As an alcoholic, I had let it control me for twenty-two years, and yes, I got lost in it. I was angry at how it took my life, took my resources. Anger should be directed toward the source, and so I hated alcohol for what it: could, would and did do, not only for what it has done;—but I came to the realization—it is I who cannot use it, not the other person, for maybe they can use it, and if so I should not be angry at them, which can be a side effect. For example, my brother Mike can drink sensible, I can't. I could never understand how a person could leave a beer sit on a bar and go home. Why? I'd ask myself, why he even came to the bar unless he was going to get something out of it, like get drunk—smashed. I asked myself, "What other purpose is there?" And never got an answer, because it was so obvious to me: to get smashed, or it should be.

5) Bargaining: is another stage we all seem to have to cross before we heal in the grieving process. Like buying a car, house or something you really want, if you can't get it one way, you may possible try another, and so what do you do: you bargain it. When I was in Haiti, doing some missionary work up in the mountains, in 1986, which I found out quickly, I was no missionary, but I did help build a medical clinic for the inhabitants in the region. And Well, I liked—for the most part—to bargain, and so the group of eighteen-others, had me do all the bargaining for them. But what I am really implying is this: you have been found out, you're an alcoholic, you can't hide it anymore, and you start to think, maybe, just maybe I can try to: "Control my Drinking," that might work, when you've endlessly tried and have not been able to stop. You bargain for another try, but you got to dump that bargaining in the garbage can, you can never use safely…period. And you may want to ask the question: why would you want to, after your substance usage took all it did from you?

6) Depression. When my mother passed on, the nurse asked, if I was depressed, I said, "I don't think so, but I'm very, very sad." She took that possible for being depressed, and maybe I was. I had come to the conclusion, with my mother; there was nothing that could be done. She died after 24-days in the hospital at 82 ½-years old, with some complications. Basically, old age; I share this because we get sad. Depression on one hand is a disorder, and was this what the nurse was talking about? I don't think so. But being very, very sad, may have a connotation of a momentary depression, and what does a person do in this area you go back to drinking often times. You go back to what you know best, what will solve the hurt, thinking it will take care of the problem, when you feel, nothing else can. So she and my doctor was very worried, and for good reason. You see, my anger

didn't work anymore, I couldn't bargain any longer; I was once again, powerless, what I had learned 22-years previously, concerning alcohol, which was of course, that I was powerless. Like my mother's concern over my healing 22-years ago, so the nurse and doctor's concern was over my starting back up again…as it affected my wife. But I didn't, thanks to everybody;— we are not islands, we need people; and again I thank the nurse, my doctor, my wife, and my mother. And I think my brother was a little concerned so thanks to him, in his silent, poised way.

7) Acceptance. If we go through the whole gamut of emotions, and healing we should run into acceptance along the way. Please remember, everybody grieves differently, some longer, some not so long. Some cry more and heal faster; others are more logical, and acceptance comes quicker. Some people are angrier, and it takes longer. Some keep bargaining. Again, whatever floats the boat. And a loss is a loss; a death of a relationship is just that, a loss. No matter if it was a mother, or alcohol. Anytime we let go, give a part of our life up, we will create stress, this is called the grieving process. If you are not willing to let go, as an alcoholic or addicted person, and remain in that role, of course you will not recover, it is plain and simple, you will not go forward in life, and die an early death. Acceptance never asks if you like it, it only tells you, to accept it.

Well, we made it through another chapter, short as they may be, if you are thinking about having a spouse go to Aftercare with you, or are in an AA or support group, or you simply need to deal with emotions, it might be wise to get more material on these steps, work them. A loss is a loss, in your search for a decision, may God be with you and give you strength. Now for the next chapter, number #4.

4

First Things First

If you want to drive across the desert
You do two things: first you kill the
Scorpions; second you build the roads.

Likewise, if you want to recover: first
You stop your usage—second, you build
A personal program [a plan: and work it].

Simple: Dlsiluk

Relapse Prevention, Recovery Topic [s]

The guts of Aftercare is right here, right upon us—yes, it is the primary topic of this book, the center, where without it, there would be no Aftercare. Relapse Prevention, is the bones to recovery. A good relapse prevention plan [which is equivalent to a program], will help you immensely through the trials and tribulations that lay ahead. It can be the difference between life and an early death. Most alcoholics die in their 40's believe it or not; and drug addicts never get old, unless that is when they start their usage. Every Aftercare program has to have some kind of structured in, Relapse Prevention that is; tied into their Aftercare program. If they do not, I'm not sure what to call Aftercare, for it would not be part of what I'd call the Continuum of Care. Put another way, part of the Continuum of Chemical Involvement.

Before we get too deep into *Relapse Prevention*, let me just hit a bit on Chemical Involvement for you. We really have an assortment of categories in this area; such as 12-which I know of. But instead of presenting the levels for you, what really matters is what we are dealing with. Let me try to summarize this if I can.

Chemical Involvement:

[For your information]

People are different, in that, people's involvement with chemicals takes on a different perspective, or point of view, by looking at their involvement. In Aftercare this is not the major concern, in that, it should be history now, but on the other hand, it is a concern to see where the person is at. If you are in what I call the first five stages, which deals with *Total Abstinence*, meaning no use at all: at the level of *Risk Use*, meaning you are starting to demonstrate, or exhibit some behavior of chemical abuse or pathology, is quite different than the next two stages, being 5 & 6, which indicate *Episodic Abuse* or *Situational Abuse*. What you are telling me [or what I am seeing is] is that you are more involved with chemicals, and this is what will help me to help you. In stages 5 & 6, you are really telling me [in my analytical mind], you are using irresponsible or having problematic chemical use; yet it may be time-limited to up to six moths of irresponsible use. Possible indicating a death in the family provoked this, or something else.

Now, when we go to the next level, stages: 7 & 8, we are entering another zone, if you will: these areas are called *Chronic Abuse*, and *Chemical Dependency*;—possible meaning, continual, or life-long misuse. In essence, you are suffering, and have a pathological relationship with mood-altering chemicals. You have an illness.

The last three stages are Early, Middle, and Late stages of Chemical Dependency. I need not elaborate, but let me say for safe keeping, harmful consequences: social, emotional, physical are in motion, and insanity is at the end of the road. Now let's head on over to Relapse Prevention.

Note: by the counselor knowing what level or stage you were at [the client], while in Aftercare, he can have some kind of awareness of your potential need, that is to say, he can be more sensitive to your recovery process. A person who was diagnosed as being in a Chronic Stage of usage, might need more care or attention, or possible direction to other resources of treatment, or aware of the recourses at his or her disposal/retention, than say, someone who was more a problematic user only.

Relapse Prevention [and Recovery]

In my previous book, "A Path to Relapse Prevention," I capitalize on, of course, Prevention for the most,—in Aftercare, Prevention is one element in the program, and so I will not put all that much time into this area. But let me briefly outline the dynamics.

To understand Relapse Prevention, you must understand how it comes about—otherwise it will not make sense; and it should. It does not start with the first drink; it is really a dynamic of an element already reactivated. It is not by chance you ended up at the Gem Bar, at 9:30 PM, on Saturday night, 1999, just when Sam and Harry were there, and *happy hour* was at its peak. No, no, something else happened. Reactivation comes in the form of a pattern you once knew or triggered by denial, isolation, stress, impaired judgment.

Have you ever heard the man say: "I just can't figure it out, what got me started again?" In most cases I could or would say, "Man oh man, just open up your eyes, trace your last week of events and you will see why you're at the Gem Bar," or Harry's or the Mont-airy Bar. No big secrets here my friends, it should be loud and clear. But instead of me making you feel bad, let's look at where it was created from: that is, let's look from a different view.

What Really Happened?

Most counselors don't even know this, so if you are a recovering alcoholic, you will be wise beyond the knowledge of the helper, in most cases that is. What, I mean what really happened to provoke this relapse. Why didn't he see it, or prevent it. And it is not because he didn't attend my classes, if that is what you are thinking. I'm not that egotistic. But there are good reasons to look at. And it is sad. I had a relapse and I suffered dearly for it. I stopped drinking to save my marriage, and it didn't get saved, and I started back up for another three years [after a year of sobriety]. And did I ever make up for lost time.

But let's look at the dynamics, the motivation to go back into hell's waters. We are not going to look at the surface, but under the surface, that is where the problem is: fear and uncertainty, had gripped the person, in most cases. A lack of confidence crept into the person's mind, not feeling the ability to stay sober: that is why, when someone uses in treatment, I get rid of those folks quick, because they can infuse this into the group [or a group, per se, that being a lack of self-belief to remain sober].

Now we can go backwards and look at *Denial*, which is of course, reactivated at this juncture also, it is a relapse dynamic. I was going through counselor school and after my divorce, started using, yes, denial crept in. I had to stop my schooling, it was not conducive. Another thing that was present in many of my classes that provoked a relapse was that, when someone would tell me, "I'm stopping drinking, and that is that," they felt they did not need Aftercare anymore, and that it was a waste of time. Down the road, was a bar from my office, and after work I'd spot their cars in the bar parking lot. Of course they were dismissed if they were using, some did stop for a coke, in essence, to see if they could walk into a bar and not use; all these little tricks. This is another reason why I do not like to force or impose sobriety on anyone, if they do not want it, then they need more pain, and there is enough out there for a life time, and I had enough, and need to help people, that want help.

For a person to attempt to stop using he needs to make a private judgment, ruling may sound better, to himself, first, not to me. The issue of sobriety has got to be worth his time, to make it worth my time. He has got to see sobriety is a better way of life than using, if he cannot see this, why in heaven's name he would stop. You got to offer this person something better, and if we counselors cannot do that, we better get out of the business. But on the other hand, all we can do is offer, and if he has not made this verdict, to deal with the issues of sobriety, then no matter what we offer is simply not good enough.

Relapse Dynamics

If you are looking at what is happening to yourself, or your spouse, in the relapse area, you might want to look for: defensiveness, or rigid behavior patterns arising; or compulsive behaviors starting up again; or tendencies toward loneliness; or are you, or your client, or your spouse who is recovering, forming 'Tunnel Vision," that is to say, focused exclusively on or in one area, avoiding all other areas? Obsession may prove to be a mirage of security and safety, for the potential relapse victim. Is wishful thinking filling you head, instead of life planning? That can be a cue; how about lack of objectives or too much daydreaming again, back to the wishful-thinking area.

For the individual:

Other dynamics you may want to look at are: feeling hopeless, that nothing can be solved. Do you feel in an immature state of happiness? Or is there a lot of confusion in your head, and has it increased in the thinking area for awhile? Irritation with friends can be a signal something is up. Are you easily angered, and for no reason? Often times before a relapse, over-reaction takes place. Are you eating well balanced meals [you are what you eat]? How is your sleeping [insomnia can be a signal]? One may get the inability to sleep, by over-sleeping. Now look at this with an open mind. When people are first recovering, they sleep a lot; and if they have an illness attached onto their recovery, they could require more sleep than normal; I am not referring to these areas.

For you:

Do you get periods of depression? if so, you most likely have a tendency for isolation, irritability. While working in the hospital, many of my clients fit this description. Depression can become more severe and frequent, and needs to be watched.

Are you cutting out your regular attendance meetings, or treatment meeting, or Aftercare meetings, or AA meetings: this sporadic dynamic, can be another cue of a potential relapse in the making; along with the "I don't care," attitude, and self-pity. Let me describe my version of self pity: it is when someone can help themselves, and pretend they can't; the syndrome, '…feel sorry for poor little me.' If you are not in a wheelchair, and you can walk, you do not need my pity, but a kick in the ass to get you moving. Perhaps, you can learn how to kick yourself in the ass, I can actually do it, try it once.

Oh I could go on all day in this area, but I need to get on to other areas, but what we are talking about is, "Loss of Control." Yes my dear friend, the ability to control was lost along the way, and sometimes you don't even see it. I know I've been hard on you here, but alcoholism, or going back to drug usage, is not a way to get control, you will have it if you do not pick up that bottle, or use that drug, then my friend, control is in your pocket.

5

A Checklist for Hidden Anger

It has been said: men release anger, and hide hurt, and women hide anger and release hurt. True or not, it boils down to this [like it or not]: hurt and anger are relatives. If you have a lot of anger, underneath that is hurt; if you have a little anger and a little hurt, you most likely have worked on hurt [which is good]; if you have a lot of hurt and no anger—you need to ask why? for there should be some. Yes, these feelings must be worked out, released, dealt with, or they will come out sideways, like it or not. In recovering people: drugs, alcohol, gambling, etc, there is an assortment [or one could say abundance] of both: anger and hurt—more than enough—to go around, normally, for everybody. And so, in **Aftercare** you have a good chance to work on what is left. That is to say, you should have worked on it prior to Aftercare, and this should just be a checklist for you, or a slight adjustment. In essence, taking your inventory, which again should have been dealt with in treatment, can affirm whatever adjustment you may need. So having said all this let's look at the list:

1. Got unnatural pain in the stomach?

2. Depression, too much sadness for your normal self? That is to say, unrea-sonable sadness…being sad is not bad in itself; it is a form of recovering. I was sad when my mother died, almost went into depressions, and possible I did. But sadness should say, "You had good times with her." When we get into depression as a disorder, that formula will not work anymore.

3. Unnecessary tightness in the face especially during your sleeping hours or resting time.

4. Inadvertent body movements?

5. Fatigued when you should be rested?

6. Irritability over little things? Look for displaced anger, that is, your anger at something or someone other than it should be; and/or taking it out on something you are not angry at. Maybe you need to direct the anger at what you're mad at.

7. Boredom, why? Why should you be loosing interest in things; that is your question, in things that you normally would not bore you? Remember grieving is a natural process and I am not trying to tell you not to grieve, but some things are not natural, and you need either education, medication, rest, prayer, talk's therapy: something. Yes, you need help or someone to help you along. When my mother died, my brother took a few trips to settle his nerves. For myself, I went to the doctor, talked to people, finished a book "A Path to Relapse Prevention," and a sort of other things to console myself during this process, and prayer. It has been six months now, and it still hurts. And I think of her each day. And tears don't come as often, but they still do come now and then. And I find myself reflecting a lot about her. And so, the process is working.

    You may ask the question: did you feel like drinking…Yes, at one part of my early grieving process, right before I had seen the doctor. But that was a feeling; I did not put it into action.

8. Check out your intonations, your tone of voice. Are you speaking real loud?

9. Dreams, nightmares—how are they coming? Again, if prayer is your thing, get on your knees and find peace, find God; if it is medication, use it; if it is therapy, get it.

10. Smile. It's hard, and after my mother died, that is the last thing on this earth I wanted to do; really, I could have died. She died 6-months ago, from the writing of this sentence, and it still hurts, but I have dealt with it, and I do smile. You see, there is a time for everything on the face of the earth, and that means also there is a time for grieving to stop. Death is universal, I will die also. And so, little by little I put back on this face of mine a smile. Talked to my doctor at the VA hospital and she was very kind to me. And talked to my brother, and wife, and everyone [as I partially mentioned in the previous paragraph]; and was quiet for awhile, and again I repeat, the smile went back on. Yes, I found out I wasn't the only one in the world that lost a loved one. And I suppose it will happen again. And I have been in war, Vietnam, for a year, 1971. But never, ever was I torn apart as when my dear mother died. So if I can, you can, put the smile back on. And I know my mother would have it no other way. I have thought about her everyday since she died, and I'm

not sure if it will be everyday until I die, but if it is so, it is ok, and if it is not so, again I'm ok with that, but the smile will be there now, sometimes not so big, sometimes a little sad, but sadness, again, only reflects good times.

11. How is your humor now-a-days, sarcastic, ironic, cynical, flipped—four questions in one, why?

12. Procrastination?

Hidden Anger: This is not about rant and raving—which is anger out of control, but rather forms of anger called: irritation [as if you can not get through a door], or a hassle, as if someone or everyone is bothering you. These are simply negative feelings that seem to hold on to one common goal: sinful or unhelpful. Something that is not the norm, yet something that seems to come no matter what; sometimes the angry person doesn't even know he's angry. I think when my mother died, I didn't know, I was angry, or if I did, I wasn't' sure what to call it: I was too overwhelmed; thereafter comes damage control. Anger is neither right nor wrong, it just is, and it's an emotion. But, and this is a **Big But**, the anger belongs to you, not me, not her or him, or anyone else, it is yours my friend, the anger is yours, as well as the trigger that made you angry. Do not lay it at my foot steps; you are responsible for your own feelings.

Anger is yours as I say again, and let's not try to justify you being angry, or if you are allowed to have anger, you are allowed to have it, and you do not need to justify it, it just is. Do not say, "My feelings should be," nor let someone else say, "You should feel", point of fact, you are feeling this way, like it or not, no matter what he or she or you say. What you need to do is make a decision, create a plan, like you do with everything else. You know, like one plans to buy a house, food, or other things. One plans the needs for the car, like gas, insurance, etc. It's a process, and I know you don't like it, but tough, it is part of dealing with a situation. Do it and stop the belly aching?

What you do not want to do is: hide from it, or as it is said in the addiction field, go to: 'disassociation,' which may involve, going to gambling [a cross-addiction now], or to some other kind of addiction. You got to get it: out, out, out, out, out, out, out. Get the picture yet? Find friends, groups, therapy, pray, but you need to express. And since this is Aftercare, you need to bring it up to your counselor, or group: the End.

6

Affirmations

Everyone needs a hug, yes oh yes, and sometimes you got to do it yourself, this is how:

It is called <u>Affirmations,</u> and if your wife feels it is too much for her to see you patting yourself on the back, then tell her to do it for you: but it can work for you, and is simply another tool in the toolbox of helping the recovering person on the road to avoiding a relapse, or a slip in his addiction. When I started using these on myself in AA groups I felt funny, in a like manner, when I asked people to use them in group therapy in treatment, or in Aftercare, they felt funny. We all do, don't we? Sure we do, that is to say, we all feel funny saying: "I am a very like-able person!" Why? Maybe because we heard for so long, "I am a very incapable person?" During my recovery, I picked one out a day, along with reading the read book on the 12-steps, and a daily devotional book. In any case, let's hope your Aftercare group can figure out better ones than I can, but how about these:

I am a very funny and humorous person.

I am a person that can learn anything given the chance.

I am truly a person of quality.

I am great, I mean down-right cool, in a wholesome way.

I can say no or yes, it is not up to the other person, it's up to me.

I am an attractive person.

I am very able.

I can change.

I can grow, instead of simply go through life.

I have courage, and that means saying what needs to be said.

I have pride, but that includes needing other people also.

I am an insightful person, and kind.

God loves me, and always has, no one is perfect.

I am a valuable person.

I can be calm, and I am learning.

I think you got the picture, and I can write a book, and now I'm doing it, and it will make sense, how do I know, I'm doing it. You're reading it. If I make mistakes, I hope you forgive me, but I'm not perfect, and will not take it to heart, but will try better next time.

7

Symptoms of Chemical Dependency

1. Drug—a slanting existence [or way of life]: Often referred to as 'Psychological Dependency.' In my other two books, '...Sobriety,' and '...Prevention,' I get more into the psychological elements of the addiction. But let me point out a few things here. When drugs become more important in your life than life, you are most likely then to be as physically attached to it, as much as you are mentally obsessed by it. I have pointed out in other books, such things as a person gets to the point of: using alone, finding more occasions to use, social drugs become one's medicines, and as expected, you want to be around your kind: other drug users.

2. Psychological—I know, I've just mentioned this, let's go for round two: obsession that is where we are remaining at, thinking about it, thoughts swirl about usage. Guess: intoxication? Yes you are preoccupied with the usage of drugs, that is a symptom, what this chapter is about, in number one, when I was saying, it was becoming or became a way of life, now it is even more so, another step up, or level down, however you perceive it, it is not good: it is being absorbed by it, you are most likely hoarding it, hiding it for later, or you did. In Aftercare, what we need to do is remind you this was your past, not present, and that it could be your future; you see, we can never, ever use safely again—point blank, no questions please.

3. Emotional—Are you, or did you notice how fast you were putting those drugs down. You know you do not have to read this paragraph every week, but on occasions, it's a good reminder where you were at. Of course you were dumping them down, just like one drinks coke. How about impulsivity? How about fortified does? How about being itchy in delays in usage; yes, oh yes, you got the picture, and can probably draw me a better one.

4. Self Regard—How are we doing above? Feeling like you just left home? Oh well, you've been there, did that most likely, and if your spouse is reading

this, friend or lover who is unfamiliar with this area of concentration, sit back and relax, you can learn, or get in the way. And you really do not want to get in the way I hope; and believe it or not, some folks do, you know: like getting in the way—stopping another person's progress so they can baby-sit them: having them dependent on them. Some loved ones really, deep down inside, do not want to loose a care-taking job.

Oh well, let's proceed: do you love yourself? Do you regard yourself as ok? In my other two books on addiction, prevention and drugs, 'self-esteem,' is brought out, which of course is the same as regard and love. Same thing as saying: 'I have value,' like in our affirmations. You see, one leads into the other. Can you take a few compliments without loosing it? If not you got it my friend, the 'dead bee,' sting, that paralyzed you [shame]. Possible with a little shame mixed up in the bowl of confusion. Are you putting yourself down…NOOOOOOOOOOOOOOO, do not ever, ever put yourself down? You know what I mean? by saying such things as: "Man I am so dumb." Never, ever do that. We all do dumb things, but that does not make us dumb.

5. Stiff Unhelpful Attitudes—you know what I'm talking about? It means you're an asshole; yup, we can even add a goofball possible to this. In nice terms, it means you are not very nice. What must you do—read: be kind, be caring, be positive, and socialize with your up head normally, not stretched out and up like an ostrich, that is to say, not in the air [see now we're just going to the opposite of Self-esteem]. Change and correct yourself, before you have to, or someone makes you.

6. Defensive—now why would you want to be defensive? Protective, suspicious, the word defensive has a lot of connotations, but why? You got to ask questions, yourself questions, why, why, why, why, why…? Why are you trying to hide, protect your drug [and that includes alcohol, and gambling, and compulsive eating]? Do you want me to tell you? Or does your spouse or loved one sitting down by you, want to know? I'll tell him or her now: get up, this is for you, because I do not think the user wants to tell you this secret [this can be called denial if you want to call it that]: he/she has worked very, very hard at his/her system, years and years at it [right?]. Matter of fact, he/she has an ongoing relationship with it, the drug, just like you, but he chose the drug, you already know that though, unless things have changed. He doesn't want to divorce it.

7. Delusion—yup, we got them. But just what are we talking about. Haw, get the loved one back here; this is for them as well as you: it is called **truth**. One

of the symptoms of Chemical Dependency is the failure to look at the truth. If you did, you'd be liable. So what do we do best? Come on. Tell your loved one or the group what you do best, or did best—coward, you know what it is, what you did: you blamed others.

8.   Weakness—you cannot stop it because of weakness? Is that not right? "No," you say. Why [that damn why gets in here all the time]—Why? You have what is called powerlessness, helplessness, and hopelessness, which is truly a consequence of chemical use. If he or she is telling you, if you are still there [the none-addictive], and he is saying I will quite, that is bullshit right from the bull's door. That is a symptom.

9.   Physical—oh everything comes with the package. Today you can drink five beers and they get you drunk, tomorrow six, next year a 12-pack, and somewhere down the road, a case of 24-bears. You can do this with any alcohol drink, or drug, the progression is about the same. Along with memory failure and withdrawals and decreased tolerance, etc.

In Aftercare we should not have to worry about this so much, just remind ourselves where we were, where we are at, and where we could end up,—save for the fact, we come to the belief it could not happen to us.

8

A Few Facts:

Suicide and Death with our Youth: It is a fact, that suicide is high among teenagers in high school. It is also a fact, that suicide is high among college students; and yes, most fail in actually dying in the process, but a high percentage does not. It is a fact Indian teenagers have a high death rate. I was going to work at an Indian facility in Minnesota, but it didn't workout the way I wanted, but I did find it was an ongoing concern for the tribe whom seemed to be getting a lot of money from the casino, yet even though their lifestyle had changed financially, so did their drinking habits: they drank more, and higher quality liquor.

On another note, did you know, more black teenagers kill themselves in the Northern part of America than white teenagers; and more white teenagers kill themselves down South than black teenagers. I have lived in both the South and North, and one can see the pressures on both ends of the Mason Dixie Line.

In addition, there are more females than males committing suicides.

I worked for many years with teenagers and to be quite honest, it was hard. If only they not only had the drug and alcohol issues, but the growing pains, the self-destruction circles came along with it, and of course the drugs and alcohol. Adolescents are dying for attention, to be listened to. Half the time they don't give-a-shit what you say, they just want to be heard. Some of this has to do with the separating of families, so we cannot blame everything on drugs and alcohol. We can look at isolation as a hindrance also. Yes, they are crying for a plan, as they listen to their loud music, and eat their fast food, and write their letters, "Dear Mom and Dad…" Some 12, others 14, and you name it, and you can pick the age. So what do we do? I got the answer, but no one will like it: just don't become an adult. But you see, that is the point, or possible, they are trying to.

So as we recover, and sit in our Aftercare sessions, we also can become better parents, and let our kids know where we've been. If they don't listen, well, they will just have to suffer. But let's hope they do, as you guide them.

There is no crystal ball, no real magic wand to all this, I had five kids, and well, let me leave it at that. But I know what doesn't work, rather than what does: first, not communicating will not work; second, isolation will not work; third, drugs and alcohol will not work; forth, an overdose will, that is why they overdose. Let's skip to the fifth: he needs sleep, but not too much, and if he gets too much, he needs to get up, so we have a roller coaster here, too little vs. too much. But what am I really saying: depression vs. insomnia? Has he lost too much weight, why? Did someone he knows commit suicide? Good question.

Now let me close this area of thought, it is depressing; I am not saying suicide has gotten to some epidemic proportion, matter of fact to the contrary, but we need to look at our battle for there are many sides to it.

9

Hidden Agenda

In Aftercare, or for that matter in any group setting, let me rephrase this: in any therapeutic setting, one usually [the group leader or facilitator, the counselor] will sit on his chair, let's say we have a group and there are thirteen clients, or patients in the group, and we are in Aftercare, as this book is related to, and the counselor opens the group up. Now normally he has the group engage in what is called a few minutes of talking about their weekend, or week, etc.,—how they did, or if they had any triggers, or relapses, or close calls. In inpatient or outpatient treatment, this conversation may last for a few minutes; let's say 3 to 5 minutes. Some members may pass, and simply say: "My weekend or week was normal, no ups or downs, or surprises, no damage, no crisis, nothing out of the ordinary, to include urges to use." Now some counselors spend more time in this circular discussion than they do in the rest of the session program, let's say it is for three-to-four hours long, the treatment session that is, or for that matter, the Aftercare session. On the other hand, some counselors do not even get into having the 'hidden agenda' brought out; only want each member to say: hello, my name is…

Now, having said that, here is my—I want to say opinion, but let's say instead, my therapeutic view on the matter: let's say for the sake of this statement, you are now in Aftercare, and as such, Aftercare is an extension of the Continuum of Chemical Involvement, or Care—: that means in essence, you are working on— or should be working on—abstinence [in some few cases 'selective abstinence'];—by saying this, what I imply is: you are on a different road than when you first started, which is now called 'Non-Use,' which points to attending A.A. groups, and ancillary services, non-residential care, etc. Not Primary Prevention programs for the most part or intervention services or for that matter even treatment. Now having said all that, I would spend as much time needed in the circle of releasing a person's 'hidden agenda;' as I have indicated before, as needed, without hindering the group process. That is to say, if it did not take the whole session. Why, because that is what Aftercare is about. And I may recommend additional services if this group was not what he/she needed to handle the issues being presented.

Normally, a person will express in the group some family issues, or health issue, or decision making issues, and one's feelings that go along with them, and it is good to process them, then and there. It is pretty hard for a group to go ahead with its normal routine when members are congested with ongoing dilemmas, mixed feelings, hurts, and anger, and pain. Once this is out of the way, then the counselor can carry on with his program. Matter of fact, if the counselor has his program written out a week in advance, as I did, he can do some quick substituting, and whatever the issues are at hand, he may be able to grab a lecture on anger, or feelings, or resistance—whatever the 'hidden agenda' demands and present that to the group.

But working with the 'hidden agenda', is a super tool for the client to get it out, and go ahead with his life. To be heard, get ideas, and maybe one can not fix everything up, but once out, it will possible take the edge off the corners so he or she can sleep a little better, and in many cases, the rest of the session will go much smoother. We must remember, Aftercare demands different rules than Treatment, and can make more allowances than a rigid program, and therefore, why not work on what the client needs, and that is the 'here and now,' elements of his life.

10

Anxiety

Some alcoholics have depression, others have anxiety. In both cases they can be disorders, or learned bad behavior. In my past two books I've brought out depression more so than anxiety;—but now that you're healing, and in Aftercare, anxiety seems to be needed. I, myself had more anxiety than depression. But I worked with both during the few years I was employed at a 'Freestanding Facility,' in the dual disorder area.

Anxiety, we can call it panic if you wish. It doesn't mean you are going crazy, or that you have schizophrenia, of which I've worked with these humble folks also; for Schizophrenia is a biological, genetic disorder: whereas, anxiety problems are not. Good, we got that out of the way, now,

We have this panic inside of us, and I feel at times I'll break down because of it. Is that how you feel? used to feel?

Panicky, or anxiety cannot make you do anything you do not set your mind to do: you are nervous—is what you are, and if you make a decision to jump up and down, you most likely will do so, and if you choose to calm down and lay back for a spell, you will most likely become un-panicky. Make sense? Or is it too easy for you to digest? Your muscles are under what is called 'voluntary control', meaning, your heart is under the autonomic nervous system, and if you want to control you heart beat, lay back, calm down, you have the control valve.

Being frightened and the loss of control: remember you're in Aftercare now, not Treatment, so let's think like Aftercare people: I do not know of anyone who-ever got a heart attack because of anxiety: ok, now, the rapid heart rate you are experiencing, is simply part of the natural defensive process of the heart called, 'fight or flight response'. This is normal. It will eventually go back down to normal. Matter of fact, exercise will make the heart go faster to be quite frank.

In addition to panic, or anxiety, what may cause some discomfort also is tension in the intercostals muscles in your chest area, so let us not get that mixed up with—or mistake it for—heart disease. What I am trying to get at is: anxiety is an issue, but it may not be as big as you make it. I doubt you will faint because of it, unless you have blood phobia. Fainting is not normally associated with anxiety attacks. And yes, many alcoholics have this condition of anxiety.

Now let's face the issue: panic or anxiety attacks, and I've seen them in the facilities I've worked in, and have been involved with them, but I am no expert, but let me say: these attacks have what is called episodes, where one will start [which I have done myself on several occasions in the long, far past] to hyperventilate, consequently, low level, chronic hyperventilation. Especially when one is under stress;—I've even caught people before they fell to their knees with this anxiety. What is happening here is, or I should say, what is needed here is: raise your [his/her] level of carbon dioxide through breathing restraining; thus, making it less likely that you'll experience symptoms. Remember I said you have the control valve?

Myth: many, if not most people think, "I'm not getting enough oxygen," I used to think that all the time, and try to get more in me fast. I would guess you have too much at this point, in relatationship to the quantity of carbon dioxide. Grant you, it seems to the contrary, but it is not, believe me, you need balance my friend, that is: 'oxygen vs. carbon dioxide balance.'

Why: why me? Or I could say, why you? Good question. You know, when I got these anxiety attacks, I said: "Time to have a few good beers," and that took the edge off everything. Good reason to drink, haw? Well, it was simply one of 1000-reasons I suppose, as well as any. But we are trying to get to the: 'why,' of things.

1) Possible I was genetically susceptible to attacks. Yet this does not mean I am destined to forever to be bothered by them, for I am not, I have learned how to control them, deal with them; expect them, and avoid them.

2) Stress in life. Stressors can surely be a cause of anxiety, such as buying a house, bankruptcy, marriage, divorce, buying a car, getting or the loss of a job;—the birth of a child; also, money problems, too much or too little. Learn how to down size the problem by making it a small one, you know by saying: this is really no big thing.

3) Breathing patterns can get worse during stressful times, and here we go into hyperventilation again, but you can control these by adjusting.

4) Misconceptions: can bring on fear, which gives rise to bodily symptoms of anxiety [fear of fear], thus, this can bring on attacks.

I hope this has shed some light on anxiety, it is all I know, and for those who have this issue of ongoing anxiety, and had Chemical Dependency issues, you need to look at it closer, and deal with it, as I have. It is the polar opposite of depression, which many folks get in the CD-area. I do not mean to give medical advice; I am simply saying what I have learned in the field. You need to talk to a doctor, or mental health specialist, or research this area more and do your own individual therapy if you wish.

11

The 12-steps Steps

[Interpreted and Understood]

In my first Chemical Dependency [CD] book, "A Path to Sobriety," I touched on the 12-steps, exploring lightly the fundaments of the steps. In my second book, "A Path to Relapse Prevention," I related them to one another. And in this book, the 3rd in the series, "Aftercare, Chemical Dependency Recovery," I will try to interpret them according to their character makeup.

In an Aftercare group, normally the counselor would do a group lecture on the subject, give an assignment, and talk about it during the next session. Here I will give you a summation, it is not perfect—but the counselor needs to know if you have an understanding of the steps. In Aftercare he does not have enough time to devote to it much more than six-hours I would expect, that is why they have 12 and 16 step groups. But again I say, the counselor needs to know where you are with them, otherwise s/he might just as well talk to the wall.

Interpret and Understand

My job is to interpret; your job is to understand, ok? Ok. You may have read many books on recovery, actually there are not all that many out there, and most are so full of gobbledygook, only a Yale professor could understand, but none-the-less, if you have read books on recovery, or treatment [insure they are under-standable], most give what I consider great ideas—but many do have some off the wall dreams that are coming from someone who has not walked down the same road you and I have, and it only works in their dreams, if you know what I mean. But again, that is why I take time to read these books and ideas, and scan them with my eyes for thoughts and research; but you have right this minute in your hands a formula with my three books. Let me explain. The first book of mine deals mostly with understanding, the second deals with applying; and the third is maintenance work, as you should be doing now; and as I mentioned above, interpreting takes place in all three books [be it step work or anything in this area of concentration].

In Aftercare with the simple 12-steps we have here, we see it has remained solid with the test of time, not like these new idea books. No experimentation needed here. It has proven itself to be worth its weight in whatever you value the most. The soul, its core in AA is the 12-steps—period. It should be part of your recovery program. It is like riding a horse without a saddle or harness, should you not take it as living proof of long term recovery. A man named Bill wrote them, and we have taken from him and the experiences of his followers the gift within them, the wisdom, and kept it polished, for I have been sober for 21-years, and the steps have proven to be valuable throughout all those years. Now having said all that let us get to the steps, ok? Ok.

1—We admit to God we are powerless over alcohol…that we no longer have control over our drinking. Meaning, it has control over us, that is why we say we can stop, but we continue to use. You become a slave to it.

Remember in the beginning of the book the saying, dealing with 'Denial:'

"Alcoholism is the only disease that tries to convince you that you don't have it."

2—Came to the belief that a power greater than ourselves could [can] restore us to sanity. The step is implying you are crazy. But it also implies, hope can be grabbed onto, or the promise of hope is present.

3—Made a decision to turn our will and lives over to the care of God as we understand Him, In essence, we are letting go, and so we can go forward.

But again let me quote from the beginning of the book, that as recovering person we need to remember, 'Alcohol is patient; it will wait forever for us to return to it.'

In short, all three steps 1, 2, and 3 are God steps, also known as control steps, which deal with making a decision to let go, turn it over, and grab onto hope; for you are going on a journey my comrade. I do not think Aftercare or Treatment or the 12-steps should be a hard task, and on the other hand I hope I am not oversimplifying them, but there is nothing hard here. You don't need ten books on the subject to know what to do. Now we are going to go into the *Action Steps*, the next six steps to be exact.

Action Steps

There are no hidden secrets here just plain old talk. The following steps are again action steps, meaning you have to do something to make them work for you. We have here steps: 4, 5, 6, 7, 8, and 9.

4—Make a searching and fearless inventory of ourselves [us]; you now get to 'know yourself,' who you really are; which should really be an ongoing task. Your inventory may include such things as: your strengths and weaknesses. You may want to make a list of them, and you and the group talk about those issues, if that is what they turn out to be; or you may want to bring it to the attention of your one-on-one counselor may want to talk it out with him or her; but in Aftercare, it most likely will be a group task.

5—Admitted to God, to ourselves, and to another human being...our wrongs. We call this humility. Sometimes this task may come in the form of a confrontation, or dialogue.

Again let me quote from the front of the book: "Alcoholism is the only disease that tries to convince you that you don't have it;" denial again. But you got to admit, and the demon of alcohol does not what you to convince yourself you really, truly, have it.

As steps 1 thru 3 are related, so are steps 4 and 5 related to one another. You are working on and exposing yourself in these five steps. This can be called reconciliation or 'spiritual awakening.'

Steps: 6 & 7—you are now ready to have God remove your defects [or undesirable behavior] in character, and you humbly ask Him to do so. These two steps are powerful; you are on your own now, and have to go directly to the big guy, God himself, or your higher power [whoever that is]. This is an action required.

Steps: 8 & 9—these again are two related steps, and here you make a list of the people you have harmed and you ask for forgiveness; keep in mind it is not a requirement they give it [forgiveness that is], just that you asked for it. In essence, you are trying to repair any damage previously done. I had to do this and it was most humbling at best, but you end up clearing the table of any sharp chicken bone.

Steps 10, 11, and 12, go together; they are called the maintenance steps.

In these three steps you can make and take time to review your inventory of unwanted behavior; and when you find those little 'blind spots,' things we did not see before, but see now, correct them, work on them. Remember no one is perfect, and therefore we can't expect ourselves or others to be perfect. We no longer need to hide that fact. We continue to keep our spiritual life up, alert and pray for understanding. Most of us pray, Christian, Jew, Muslim, Buddhist, Gay people, Hindu; I have been in synagogues, churches, mosques, Buddhist temples, and prayed at Hindu shrines. I have counseled gay people as well as Christian people. It is all about keeping the spirit full, when you direct it to the Creator; you are trying to talk to him. It is what we need to do, however you do it. In addition to these steps, we now need to reach out and help another person, why not, you're all fixed up now, Right?—☺ **Help fix another person up…it's ongoing my friend.**

The 12-steps are simply a recovery tool, no more, no less. It was not the beginning, nor is it the middle or the end of anything, it is something ongoing, it simply was something someone created with God's wisdom, and it works—no magic involved. Use it.

12

The Cycle of Violence

No need to have physical violence or sexual violence in our picture, but it often comes like it or not. Being 20-years in this business, and 22-years using, and 21-years chemically free, "Violence" is an unsharpened edge just waiting around every corner of a user.

In this last section, I want to bring out to the client, and counselor, the new counselor possible, or the old one that wants to bush up on old things a few dynamics in the area. We as growing, and un-using clients, need to keep our balance, likewise we need to take our inventory, and let us not forget, be kind. In doing all these things, which help us stay in check, some of us having that wild streak in us yet need this more than others, and yet some may not even need to review this at all. But here we go:

1) First of all, let's define Violence;—how about "Power and control."

2) Now we are on our way. Making and carrying out threats this is violence? We can look at it in a few different ways. If you are a landlord—and you are a woman—and a tenant threatens to hurt you if you do not let him do this or that, this is violence. On another level, a child may tell a parent, I'll commit suicide if you do not do this or that. Again, we are dealing with using coercion and threats to get our way. I have been involved in both such cases with clients. Also, "I'll report you to the Welfare, or the IRS, if you don't do this or that." Another threat is: "Drop charges or *else;*" which normally the *'else'* means: I'm going to hurt you like I've been doing right along.

3) Using Intimidation: how about those looks, and actions, gestures. Are you getting your control by using them, I did that once to an old man and women when I was using alcohol, I was only 15-years old. I looked at the old man and woman with evil eyes, and I continue to remember his frightened face to this day. I wish I could have taken that back, but that was 40-years

ago. I also smashed things when I was temperamental, after a drinking spell, or getting drunk, not hurting anyone per se, or physically, yet, if you stood by watching, it was intimidation. I have *had* friends, who abuse pets when under the influence of drugs and alcohol, and had a few used weapons, in one case a friend of mine died by a weapon—got shot.

4) Using Emotional Abuse: we do normally use all we can—do we not? [That is, to get the power and control.] And to be quite honest, we are creative. You know, like belittling her, or not allowing her to see or talk to anyone, or timing her as she goes to 'Target,' yes oh yes. I had a female friend's husband do that, and in so doing, my friend was intimidated, and it is called: control and this control is called: Violence. I often used a more psychological approach to get my way: make them feel guilty. One of my wives used to play mind games that are emotional abuse. Humiliating a person, or shaming somebody—both the same, is a sin. So if you are in Aftercare reading this, you might want to take note, and see if you are still doing any of these things, if so, get back to reality jerk, you don't own anyone, no one.

5) Using Seclusion: this is a good one. A family member continues to do this, that is, he or she goes on with doing this seclusion thing, and it works: the person uses it to control his wife, his kids to the point of no return: meaning, controlling what she does, who she sees, talks to, where she goes; in addition, he forbids her to do things without his permission, as a result, limiting her involvement with other people in the outside world—why? Again to insure she does not get too far away from him so he can do with her mind as he pleases. Often times, he doesn't even know she's being cooked alive until she is.

6) Responsibility—I want to work with the words: 'reducing and denying:' what I am really saying, by saying this is—to the world outside our mind, also to our family in particular—we are not serious, not taking things somberly: implying, as if this [something] or that [something] really didn't happen. Saying she, or they caused it—blaming. What we are trying to sew together is taking responsibility; you like to take your rights: right? So also one must learn to take one's responsibility.

7) I've been married a few times, and have children, five to be exact. And one of the power-control areas a lot of people use is: children. I have done many things wrong in my life, but I have not used children to get my way. And in two marriages, it is sad to say, they have. Like so many others out there. And the courts do little or nothing about it. Judges are as fickle as the abusers are

abusive. They do not look at what is written anymore, they for some odd reason, think they got it in their heads, and make personal judgments that do not help the child. I have seen this in the Courts of St. Paul, Minnesota for 20-years, and in the courts of Columbus, Ohio. It is a down right sin, and these judges, and especially referees [that think they are judges] should be thrown off the benches, and out of the courtrooms of America. You see, even judges and referees can abuse power, and they do. But let's look at this a little more. Abuse or using children comes into play when we use visitation to hurt or trouble the other person, or threatening to take the children away. Allowing a family member to be deprived of the child because the mother wants to sail to Florida or move to Washington, something like that, and takes the child with her. That is using the child. Then the judges wonder why parents are angry and mad, and children are spoiled, and people get hurt. The judges do it as does the legislature in most every state; my beautiful St. Paul, Minnesota being the worse of the lot. And this goes for everything, especially if you're in the Landlord business; get out of it if you're in St. Paul.

8) Male Privilege, female advantage: threatening one another as if that person is a servant. Not just males, no, no, let's add females to the list. In this new modern day and age, the master of the house is not the father, and sometimes not the mother, rather the damn spoiled kids [again, a down right shame in St. Paul, Minnesota]. The male, is but the seed, with a little emotional support, and the courts trying to grab the paycheck from the male. You say a little biased, no, just truthful.

9) Financial mistreatment: let's say it is, or means 'providing;' now two people are guilty here. I know the females want to say, this is a man area, bullshit. Not any more. He gets a job, he pays his support, and the female judge says: she can move anyplace in the country with the five year old kid. Now where is the mistreatment here? The father has a home, a job, and if he wants to see the kid, he got to go where she is. And like it or not, he has to pay support. Now let's change this a bit, they are married, and living together, and she is taking care of the child, and he gives her an allowance, and she starts working, and he takes her money, and in both cases she does not know about, or have any access to bank accounts, or family income: he's an asshole [we got them in Minnesota also].

13

Recovery

Talk to other recovering people and hear what works for them. Stock up on everything you can on recovery-or recovering, as you wish. Make your sobriety—recovery a trip to enjoy. If need be, allow yourself to become the kid inside of you, but be grateful to the people willing to share with you their journey, or testament.

Now as you look back, remember what you left behind you. Possible a hospital for treatment, or clinic, and even a 'detox,' center thereabouts. Then there are the family members who had to endure, deal with your issues, a few groups of people here and there possible. Not much glimmer haw? But a lot of hard work to get where you are now; but then that is part of recover, work.

Possible your road to recovery has been 30 to 90 days; or a year, or two or three—being sober that is. Mine is 21-years, but then it has had it bouts also. But we keep on trucking, moving on. When I got my three year medallion, I thought I had really earned it, and when I got my eight-year medallion, I was so proud, now I've never got another one, not sure why. But just writing this third volume is making me think about getting one.

When you first went for help, stepped into, or underneath the recovery Canopy, I doubt you were in any kind of good shape, physically or mentally. People rarely are. And so, you had to adjust, psychologically without your sidekick, that being, your drug of choice. But now that is behind you, now you can sleep and eat normally like other human beings. Now that lead me into what I want to talk on for a quick moment:

Sleep. Sleeping sober was one of the greatest gifts I was given for my sobriety, or so I feel. Most non-addicted folks do not realize how we suffer for sleep. And normally the first three months of sobriety, during this recovery stage, we sleep a lot. One time I slept 19-hours [that is right], nineteen long, long hours; what a stretched out, marvelous sleep. Matter of fact, I slept long hours for the first nine-months; forget this 90-days stuff. And thereafter for about three years I had nothing but great long sleeps, where I'd sleep about 9.15 hours per night. Man O man, did I enjoy.

Now there was a second thing I was talking about in a few paragraphs above, it was right after sleep I think, called eating. Yes eating sober is a delight. It is a gift to be able to at last taste the food, smell it; we learn that the gift, so taken for granted by others, is overwhelming for us the first few years of recovery. But of course this is our past, right; it is nice to look back and see where we came from, where we are at, and where we are heading.

I mentioned sleeping, eating, but I left out one thing, and it is called celebration. The recovery process should be a celebration; especially during the first three to eight months of your recovery. When for instance, we go through all these new feelings we forget we had, and now are discovering. Yes they are appearing on all sides of us, unpadded and fantastic at the same time. Yes, we may get some anxiety my friend, it may creep into your soul, your character, but don't let it stop the celebration. Once I saw a woman who needed to get something out, and she was so ridden with anxiety, she had to sit down, looked me in the eyes, looked at her hands shaking, and then sat on them, and started talking as if nothing was a problem. I love it, what more can you ask for. She didn't let the anxiety control her; she stopped the action before it went overboard.

Can you remember going to your first group meeting? Be at AA, NA, or a 12-step group, or whatever group, support group that is, you attended? Or any group for that matter to deal with drug or alcohol issues. At one time this AA group I am referring to, in my mind was an isolated and non-applauded club for weak people. Now I was more significant in the world when I recovered, and it was for me, and now I became comfortable with it. You see, all in time. Yes, in time the meetings became less baffling. It all means you've been on the road to recovery: as you may now be in Aftercare, which is part of that road.

Another element of the recovery process understands the main fundamentals of the 12-steps. You see, it gives a person a clear message of hope and urgency, and yes it is God-based, but it does not mean you have to be converted to anything other than sobriety. In all my 12-step work in groups no one was ever criticized at any time, or at any level for not making a commitment on talking to God; only for not taking a commitment for recovery. Pray as you will, or don't pray at all, but remain sober. Admit and be honest, this is the program in a nutshell.

The Paradox: we all should know it: Right? There is supposed to be one anyways, or so I have heard. Let me see if I can untie it, or for that matter even find it. I never had a hard time with it, but some folks do. Let me see if I can sum it up, and then tell you what they call the paradox: you don't have to act on your feelings—that's it. Now let me name it: Letting go. You may be saying this is so simple: yes and no. I made it simple, but I can make it hard. Let me give you an example: "You said to let go and I did, and I got drunk. Now this is because you told me to, so it is your fault." You ever hear that before. What the person did and didn't do was this: he was most likely trying to work the program, and as it says: 'Let go,' but forgot the last three words, 'Let go, *and let God.*' Now I said you do not have to fight with the 12-steps over God, so I left it out, as do most of the people who get caught up in this paradox. If you leave out God, you got to put in: you don't have to act on your feelings. And that is exactly what that man did. He left out the last three words, and left out feelings vs. actions. You do not act on feelings, you act on thinking. And in recovery, the recovering person may have a hard time distinguishing between 'Feelings,' and 'Thinking.' But let me straighten that out for you also: feeling is an emotion, and thinking is an opinion, idea, a thought. Now let's end this recover with a paragraph that suits this book.

Make your recovery a positive experience, by doing so you will need to have gratitude, to whoever/whatever helped you on the way, be it your mother, God, your counselor, a camel, a duck or a carrot. It doesn't matter. Gratitude is simply thankfulness. Plus you are saying: I didn't do it alone, and now you are not alone, and shall never be alone again. Now I could go on endlessly with recovery information, but let me simply say it all boils down to success, and success in this area is simply managing your sobriety. Good luck.

Afterword

Well, we're at the bottom of the book. I wasn't going to write this third volume, until I found out there really weren't any Aftercare books out there to speak of. So here is one, short and to the point. It is not a thick one; book that is, because I have only touched on the surface of what is needed. And it was not written for the Psychologist, or Doctor, yet it might help both of them. It was written for the recovering. As all three of my books were, or have been;—so, having said that, let me sum up this experience, this book:

Aftercare is an element of Primary Prevention, a part, component, I said, no more. It also is a part of, or piece of: Relapse Prevention. In addition to this, we are really dealing with—as I've mentioned before—'The Continuing Care cycle,' in which there should be an ongoing evaluation of your progress, and recommendations thereof, and objectives to go forward with. Aftercare should be more supportive than therapeutic, and to be quite honest, I really doubt you need a licensed or certified counselor to run the group, but if this is possible, so be it, and all the better for it, but surely not necessary. What you need to hear is alternatives for using. If I could not offer my clients something better than using, why stop, why would they want to stop? The process is growth. So read, meditate, do your inventory, talk to someone about your urges, get them hidden agendas out, get educated, go to lectures if need be. Get into a discussion group if need be, and use your affirmations. And make sure you give yourself a break—you deserve it.

About the Author's Books

Poetry:

Recently the author has put together a second poetry book together, one that drapes all his poems under one banner: put into newspapers, anthologies, and books since his first volume of poetry published in 1981, called, "The Other Door." This second volume, "Sirens," complements his first. And may be his only book of poetry ever to be produced again [2003].

The Tales of the Tiamat:

This is a trilogy, consisting of "The Tiamat, Mother of Demon," the second book, "Gwyllion, Daughter of the Tiamat," and the third, "Revenge of the Tiamat". All three are full of adventures and travels by Sinned, the main character of the three novels, as is the Tiamat involved, yet we see many other antagonists along side of her. The series take you to Malta, Easter Island, ancient England, and Avalon, where the Tor was being built, Asia Minor, where Yort is, Sinned's home, and a half dozen other places. In addition to the main three stories, the author has added a forth, short book to the series, called "The Tiamat and the King," it is a good conclusion to the trilogy, and put into a forth book called, "Tales of the Tiamat."

The Chick Even's Sketches:

In this trilogy, we have sketches of life that incorporate the late 60's to the early 70's; the hippie generation, the new era, the awakening of Aquarius, the peace era, it has been called many things. In his sketches, his first book: "Romancing San Francisco [1968-69]," he introduces us to karate's famous Yamaguchi family, to include Gosei, and his father Gogen "The Cat"; along with the famous Adolph Shuman, the once owner of the line of cloth Lilli Ann, along with other sketches. In the other two books: "A Romance in Augsburg," and "Where the Birds Don't Sing," the sketches start where the first book left off, from 1969 to 1970 and to Vietnam in 1971. Here you go to Europe for a Romance with a Jewish German girl, and on to Vietnam where there is a war going on. Mr. Evens will also end up in Sydney, for one week of some great adventures.

Short Story Collection [s]:

This is not a trilogy, rather three books, of which two are similar, that being of Suspense, "Death on Demand," of which there are seven stories and "Dracula's Ghost", having nine; and the third book, being a mixture of short stories, called "Everyday's An Adventure".

Spiritual:

The Author has some strong religious and spiritual views. Having studied and done graduate work in theology, and missionary work in the mountains of Haiti, and being at an earlier age an Ordained Minister, his two books, "The Last Trumpet and the Woodbridge Demon," being his first talk about experiences of the early eighties, where he had visions concerning end time events that are coming to pass right this very moment. In his second book, "Islam, In Search of Satan's Rib," he talks about the ongoing subject terrorism on America, and the world as a whole, but in a different manner; instead of trying to figure out the mind of the Islamic-Arab, he looks at the Islamic god, and concludes it is different than the Christian and Jewish God.

Addiction:

As of this writing [Oct, 2003], Mr. Siluk is still a licensed Counselor in good standing with the State of Minnesota. He has also held international licenses in Drugs and Alcohol, and has worked for hospitals and clinics in dual disorder facilities. In his book, "A Path to Sobriety, the Inside Passage," the author has used his experience in the behavioral science and counseling skills in producing it, which is a common sense book on understanding alcoholism and addiction, an ultimate guide to substance abuse; and his 2nd book, "A Path to Relapse Prevention," is a powerhouse for preventing relapse and curing the disease. In his third book, "Aftercare, Chemical Dependency Recovery," Mr. Siluk completes his three volumes with the supportive elements the recovering needs in his continuum of care.

Travels:

Mr. Siluk has travel, or has been traveling I should say for 37-years out of his 55 ½ years of his life to this date. He has traveled 25 ½ times around the world. And in most of his books you can see, feel and almost taste this [to be more exact, he has 613,000-air miles, not to include ground miles]. In his book, "Chasing the Sun," he takes you to a variety of places, by showing you some 40-pictures, and giving you an overall view of his story on how he got started. Each picture has its own caption; furthermore, this book is a page turner, for a would be traveler, or one who would like to reminisce.

The Beast Books:

I wasn't sure what to call these three next separated books, so I named them, "The Beast Books," for in their own way, they all have their own beast. The first book being, "Mantic ore: Day of the Beasts," which is the author's favorite of the three, you step into the demonic underworld. A lot of him is in this book it seems. A touch of Vietnam, a touch of his home town, St. Paul, Minnesota, and invisible shadows that change shapes into animals and human forms; visions upon visions. In the second book, the "The Rape of Angelina of Glastonbury, 1199 AD, you are involved with a suspenseful story of revenge, and at the end of the book is a nice surprise, another story. And for the third beastly book, "Angelic renegades & Rephaim Giants," you get just that, no more, no less. It is a book on the ancient dictators of the world, the ones who have cursed God, to have man worship them.

"The Mumbler:"

Which is a psychological thriller novel, I wasn't sure where to put it in these brief descriptions of books, so it will have to be alone, as the character in the book is—right here.

Out of Print book:

For the curious reader; although they are out of print, the author has a few left in storage. "The Other Door," was his first book published, in l981; a book on poetry. It is a Volume one, of which he is working on Volume two, yes, 22-years in the making. This book is so scarce that only 25-copies are left. Second, is the author's book, "The Tale of: Willie the Humpback Whale," which got much attention in the l982. Although it did not get a Pulitzer Prize, it was an entry, and considered. At present the author is considering a 4th printing, and revised edition. And the third book, "Two Modern Short Stories of Immigrant Life," which is more of a chap book that came out in l984 as a trial run. Only 100-copies were printed, of which one of the stories were printed in the: "Little Peoples Press," and then the book was pulled back for personal reasons and off the market by the author.

Visit my web site: **http://dennissiluk.tripod.com** you can also order the books directly by/on: **www.amazon.com www.bn.com www.SciFan.com www.netstoreUSA.com** along with any of your notable book dealers.

0-595-30868-6